Is Your Pet Safe?

Morgellon's Disease-A New parasitic
disease may be transmitted by pets

Neelam Taneja-Uppal, MD

iUniverse, Inc.
Bloomington

Is Your Pet Safe?

iUniverse books may be ordered through booksellers or by contacting:

iUniverse
1663 Liberty Drive
Bloomington, IN 47403
www.iuniverse.com
1-800-Authors (1-800-288-4677)

ISBN: 978-1-4502-7507-1 (sc)
ISBN: 978-1-4502-7508-8 (ebook)

Printed in the United States of America

iUniverse rev. date: 12/10/2010

ABOUT THE AUTHOR

Dr. Neelam Uppal, has had many years of experience in Infectious Diseases and internal Medicine. Dr. Uppal graduated from Christian Medical College in India. From there she went to New York where she did her internship and then did her Residency in New Jersey in Internal Medicine. She then did her fellowship in Infectious Diseases in New York hospital of Queens and Memorial Sloan- Kettering medical Center. Dr. Uppal is board certified in Infectious Diseases, on the Advisory Board of National Morgellon's Foundation, Winner of American College of physicians award in 1990, was quoted in new York Times and several National Television Shows., recently on Rachel Ray show on July 23,2010.

AWARDS AND HONORS:

- PHYSICIAN OF THE YEAR –2006 BY NRCC
- MADISON'S WHO'WHO
- STANFORD WHO'S WHO
- AMERICAN COLLEGE OF PHYSICIANS RESEARCH AWARD- FIRST PLACE-1990

MEMEBERSHIPS:

- <u>AMERICAN COLLEGE OF PHYSICIANS</u>
- INFECTIOUS DISEASE SOCEITY OF AMERICA
- FLORIDA INFECTIOUS DISEASE SOCEITY OF AMERICA
- AMERICAN MEDICAL ASSOCIATION
- FLORIDA MEDICAL ASSOCIATION
- PINELLAS COUNTY MEDICAL SOCEITY
- FLORIDA ASSOCIATION OF PHYSICIANS FROM INDIA
- AMERICAN ASSOCIATION OF PHYSICIANS FROM INDIA
- PINNELLAS PARK CHAMBER OF COMMERCE

OVERVIEW

The book is based on my practice of Infectious diseases and discovery of a new parasitic disease referred to as Morgellon's Disease. My experience made me realize the dilemmas of the recognition of the disease in the medical community and social implication. It made me understand how it may be spreading in United States and how it may be prevented as a Public Health issue. Hence to bring this awareness to the public and healthcare providers I was compelled to write this book.

A 40 years old woman comes to my office with sores all over body. Complains of crawling sensations and itching. States she sees threads coming out of her body. She grabs the hand sanitizer and rubs on her belly and tries to bring out stuff. She has been diagnosed with 'delusional parasitosis'. But in talking to her she is an extremely intelligent woman. So I decide to investigate and what I have discovered is in this book.

TABLE OF CONTENTS

CHAPTER I
INTRODUCTION

A 32 years old woman came to my office with her husband. Her face and arms were covered with scabs. She was crying. She had been checked by several doctors and was told "she was 'CRAZY'." I saw her and realized that was not true. She was sick. And she said "believe me I am sick"

She had been admitted to several psychiatric hospitals and was put on several antipsychotic medications with no relief. I admitted her in a community hospital and started her on treatment. Patient's symptoms started to resolve. I had a covering doctor on the weekend, who was a board-certified infectious Disease physician, she came and saw the patient and diagnosed her with 'Delusional Parasitosis ' and called for a psychiatric consult. When I came to see the patient on Monday morning I was told that the patient had signed out AMA (against Medivcal advise)

That led me to write this book is that I can educate the people with the disease, their families and caretakers that have to deal with these patients and the health care professionals that are looking for some answers unraveled a mysterious Disease, that has baffled the smartest of physicians. See how the pets can transmit parasites which may not be identified by your healthcare provider, and you could be deemed 'DELUSIONAL'

A woman in her forties comes to my office with sores and itching and feeling crawling sensations on her skin. The husband is ready to divorce her because she keeps acting 'Crazy' trying to show him bugs coming out of her. But he sees nothing. The patient is deemed 'Delusional'. But I realized what the patient was feeling due to her parasitic involvement and calmed the husband. The patient is now feeling better.

CHAPTER II
EPIDEMIOLOGY

That is the areas in United States where this is occurring the most and why?

Most patients that were seen were coming from California, Texas and Florida. The common things in these places are the weather, which is tropical. It is hot and all these states are on the water. This provides the environment for the organisms to thrive.

Secondly, nearly all the patients have either pets or exposure to pets or travel to third world countries or are immigrants. Some of them may have a past history of an infestation in their country.

IMMIGRATION:

Parasites are prevalent in the tropical climate third world countries. With a lot people migrating from these countries, the parasites came with them. May be their pets got infested. The pets go outside and sometimes even eat off the road another dogs' feces. A lot of people clean the litter of the cats.

TRANSMISSION:

How do Humans get this disease?

On retrospective analysis it was fund that ball patients had one thing in common that is, pets. And the pet was either sick or had worms that were treated.

The review of the life cycles of most of the parasites in the pets shows that the pets ate the intermediate host of most of the parasites.

The hot weather supports the optimum temperature for the proliferation of these organisms.

Also the availability of the water helps in the transmission of the larval stage.

For example, if the dogs had worms, he did his thing and cleaned himself, but the eggs could have stayed on. And then the owner slept with the dog, had the dog on his lap or played with the dog the eggs can get attached to the hand, get embedded in the nails and then subsequently get injected.

The water in these areas helps transmission of the larval forms. People take dogs on some of the beaches. The larval forms can get hatched and swim around and then penetrates the skin of a human being and they get the parasite.

Also the fleabites can transmit the eggs and then either deposits it in their bite or feces.

Evidence based Medicine:

The standard of practice for the diagnosis of parasites is to send stool ova and parasites under microscope.

But the regular commercial Lab Personnel is not trained. So even if you send a clearly positive specimen, the result comes back negative

When the doctor looks at the result and tells the patient that their test is negative; they do not have parasites.

And thus' the patient is labeled 'CRAZY'

CHAPTER III
PARASITES FROM PETS

There are a lot of parasites that can be transmitted by the cats and dogs.

These can be:
- Hookworm
- Tapeworm
- Toxoplasma
- Toxocara canis and Catis
- Cat Scratch Disease
- Dog Heart Worm is Dirofilaria
- Fish tapeworm- Ecchinococcus needs dogs or cats as intermediate host.
- Also called Dog tapeworm
- Pinworm
- Roundworm
- Cysticercosis, Tenia soliumm and Tenia saginatta.

- Bed bugs
- Scabies
- Resistant Scabies
- Ringworm
- Generalized rash due to Allergies

The lab results come back borderline positive. So these organisms could be related to these worms.

CHAPTER IV
NOMENCLATURE

The name of the disease

Morgellon's is referred to as Delusional Parasitosis. It needs to be corrected to unspecified Parasitosis. CDC terms it as 'Unspecified Parasitosis'

WHAT IS UNSPECIFIED PARASITOSIS:

It is a syndrome in which patients present with multiple signs and symptoms. All patients may not have exactly the same symptoms and signs.

SYMPTOMS OF UNSPECIFIED PARASITOSIS

Rash is the most common symptom. These patients have **Several** kind of **Skin Lesions.** These can be **Papules, Abscesses, Ulcers,Vesicles**

The **Organisms** cultured from the skin lesions are bacteria and fungus. They have **Thread – like or granules** come out of these lesions. These denote the larvae, the worm and the granules are the eggs. Other symptoms are Itching, Fatigue, Fever, Chills. Long term symptoms that develop are Depression, Delusions, Irritability

Published by 'Elsvier and Elsvier'

Severe nocturnal pruritus is the hallmark of scabies. Itching also may be provoked by any sudden warming of the body and generally does not involve the face. A warm bath or radiant heat may cause a paroxysm of itching. Because the pruritus is caused by sensitization, 4 to 6 weeks may elapse between infestation and the onset of severe pruritus. Re-infestation is common, because eradicating the disease from all contacts simultaneously is often difficult, and re-infestation after cure results in prompt recurrence of symptoms. Cutaneous manifestations are varied. The primary lesion is the epidermal burrow, a tiny linear or serpentine track, rarely longer than 5 to 10 mm. The female mite may burrow anywhere on the body, but sites of predilection include the interdigital spaces, palms (Fig. 44-59), flexor surfaces of the wrists, elbows, feet and ankles, beltline, anterior axillary folds, lower buttocks, and penis and scrotum. The distribution of burrows in infants may be atypical, with burrows frequently found in the scalp and on the soles (Fig. 44-60). In the present epidemic, involving many people with excellent hygiene, cutaneous changes may be almost absent and burrows difficult to find. On the other hand, after the disease has been present for some time, eczematization, lichenification, impetiginization, myriad nonspecific papules and excoriations, and even urticaria may be present. The burrows are often the least conspicuous of various skin changes. The clinical picture varies with differences in personal hygiene, topical treatments used before diagnosis, and individual scratch threshold. Scabies can also result in secondary skin cellulitis, sepsis, and postinfective complications such as glomerulonephritis. [162] [230]

CHAPTER V
DELUSIONAL PARASITOSIS

A chapter in a book published by Elsvier &Elsvier describes delusional parasitosis as

Special thanks and appreciation to Sherman Minton and Bernard Bechtel for their valuable
Patients with delusions of parasitosis are convinced, against all evidence to the contrary, that parasites infest their skin and often their homes and clothing. No single cause is known for this condition, although some cases may be associated with proven parasitic infestation. The idea may also be suggested by infestations of relatives or acquaintances. Patients older than 50 years are most often female; patients younger than 50 are equally male and female. Most cases of delusions of parasitosis commence with pruritus, which may be accompanied by crawling, creeping, stinging, and burning sensations. The initial reaction is to scratch, replaced soon by digging to remove the "parasites." Self-mutilation and suicidal behavior may develop. Generally, the first contact with a physician is to bring in evidence of the "infestation." Evidence typically

consists of scales, lint, crusts, hairs, dust, and small pieces of skin, carefully collect…

An integrated approach to personal protection is the most effective way to prevent arthropod bites, regardless of location and species. Protection from arthropod bites is best achieved by avoiding infested habitats, wearing protective clothing, and using insect repellents.[89] Insect repellents containing DEET are the most effective products on the market, providing broad-spectrum repellency lasting several hours. [89] [223] Currently available non-DEET–containing repellents do not provide protection for as long as DEET-based repellents. DEET's peak duration of action plateaus at a concentration of 50%, with no added benefit from products containing higher concentrations. [89] Additionally, liberal use of higher-concentration products with ethanol bases can lead to increased skin absorption and neurotoxicity, particularly in young children.[223] Topical insect repellents alone do not provide complete protection. Ethyl butylacetylaminopropinate (IR3535)&#x…

Oral antihistamines can be effective in reducing the symptoms of insect bites. Cetirizine was given prophylactically in a double-blind, placebo-controlled, 2-week crossover trial to 18 individuals who had previously experienced dramatic cutaneous reactions to mosquito bites.[214] Subjects given the active drug had a 40% decrease in both the size of the wheal response at 15 minutes and the size of bite papule at 24 hours. The mean pruritus score, measured at 15 minutes and 1, 12, and 24 hours after being bitten, was 67% less than that of the untreated controls. In highly sensitized individuals, prophylactic treatment with nonsedating antihistamines, such as loratadine, may safely reduce the cutaneous reactions to insect bites. [3] [226]

A 3.6% ammonium solution (After Bite) relieves the type I hypersensitivity symptoms associated with mosquito bites. In a double-blind, placebo-controlled laboratory trial, 64% of mosquito-bitten subjects exper…

Mites make up the largest group in the class Arachnida. Most are small arthropods, and many are barely visible. Mites have two body regions, a small cephalothorax and a larger, unsegmented abdomen. The cephalothorax and abdomen are broadly joined, giving most mites an oblong to globular appearance. Newly hatched larvae have three pairs of legs, and larvae acquire a fourth pair after the first molt. Mites are highly diverse. Some are parasitic, with both vertebrates and invertebrates serving as hosts; some are scavengers, some feed on plants, and many are free living and predacious. Although most species are oviparous, some are ovoviviparous, and a few are viviparous. They occur worldwide and frequently in great numbers. Mites have been associated with disease transmission, allergies, and dermatologic manifestations. Of the approximately 35,000 species, about 50 are known to cause human skin lesions.

- Delusions (seen patients, because the disease is not recognize and a lot of times patients feel the crawling, seen organisms coming out might be microscopic however the doctor's doesn't see it)** Some of the patients pull threads from a sock and when they visit the doctor they would say that it came out from their skin or on the other parts of their body. And, also because of the stress their experiencing they want the doctor to believe in them.

- Irritability – patients are irritable and anxious because they're trying to convince something to the doctor who doesn't know a thing.

The other persons who also don't know are the commercial laboratories. When I was a medical student there was a professor who used to say, " If the mind doesn't know, the eyes don't see." In this case how many lab technicians in the commercial laboratories that look at the stool specimen and knows how to identify that eggs.

It is very odd and hard to identify an egg; an untrained eye will not see it. When the result comes back it's negative. Sometimes the doctor would tell the patient that it's all in their head but no, it's more in the doctor's head who doesn't know.

I believed that why we have a lot of mis-cases happen because I don't think that the commercial laboratories were equipped enough with a trained personnel to make the diagnosis.

SYMPTOMS OF DELUSIONAL PARASITOSIS

Rash and Skin Lesions are Papules, Abscesses,Ulcers, Vesicles, Organisms that are Thread like and granules. They also complain of , Itching, Fatigue, Fever, Chills, Depression, Irritability.

OTHER SIGNS include Weight Loss – significant weight loss, Multiple Skin Lesions – in different stages, Anxiety, Swelling, Red Areas – due to Cellulitis

CHAPTER VI
DIAGNOSTIC TESTS

The other personnel who also don't know are the commercial laboratories. When I was a medical student there was a professor who used to say, " If the mind doesn't know, the eyes don't see." In this case how many lab technicians in the commercial laboratories that look at the stool specimen and knows how to identify that eggs.

It is very odd and hard to identify an egg; an untrained eye will not see it. When the result comes back it's negative. Sometimes the doctor would tell the patient that it's all in their head but no, it's more in the doctor's head who doesn't know.

I believed that why we have a lot of missed cases happen because I don't think that the commercial laboratories were equipped enough with a trained personnel to make the diagnosis. The lab results come back borderline positive. So these organisms could be related to these worms.

CHAPTER VII
LABORATORY TEST

CBC : this test should be performed to look for any signs og infections, that is, for bacterial, fungal or viral. You will see increased neutrophils in bacterial infections and lymphocytes for viral and fungal infections. You can see atypical lymphocytes for certain infections. And you may see eosinophils suggesting parasitic infestation or allergies.

Chemistry: to check for liver kidneys and electrolytes. Lymes Test should be done. Herpes Test should be done in generalized form kind of lesions

Parasite antibodies should be done. You can see cross reaction to strongyloides. Some patients have low positive reaction to Schistosoma. Echinococcus, is another test that comes out as low positive

- MRSA – (Methicillin-resistant staphylococcus aureus) detailed about the bacteriology that was presented, a lot of the times the lesion would be positive with MRSA and have not responded with any other antibiotic

Bacterial
- MRSA

- E- coli
- Pseudonomous
- Proteus

These infections were seen in these lesions, in my first opinion it was a super infection because of the skin, and the second opinion that I have that a lot of these people will have a grand negative in which is a bowel flora that is in the lesions. These bacteria were coming into the lesions because of the larva migrans from the bowel to the bloodstreams and into the lesions.

Stool O & P – I sent out samples and when the results comes in, it's always negative

Urine – patients complains that seeing lesions or stuff coming out of the urine.

I decided to examine one patient vagina because the patient told me that she found stuff on her privates. Once I open her vagina I saw a finger like white stuff crossing in front of me from one mucosa to the other. That the time I started believing that there is this disease that is called "Morgellans Disease".

ANA : I also send samples to see if there is autoimmune problem and also to look for lupus,SED rate, ANCA – is for vasculitis,

Other parasitic antibodies that are performed by the laboratories are Ankylostoma – which is the hook worm, Filaria, Dirofilaria

CHAPTER VIII
PROCEDURES

- Wound Cultures - we sent out wound cultures, which could be super infections or a suggestions where the worms coming from.

- Skin Biopsy

- Examination of parasite under microscope – patients bringing different parasite moving stuff that were sent to the lab for parasitic microscopic examination, which is usually identified as nothing or ignored or it isn't found.

CHAPTER IX
KNOWN PARASITES
DIAGNOSIS

Reported by lifescripts

{We love our pets. And when they're sick, we want to hold them close. But can they pass those diseases on to us? Yes. And some can be deadly. Find out how to keep both of you safe from the most common pet illnesses...

For many of us, pets are family. We talk to them, watch TV together, let them sleep on our beds.

But close contact can expose you to serious ailments.

That doesn't mean you should ban pets from your home. The key to keeping yourself healthy is awareness and prevention, says Margaret Lewin, M.D., Medical Director of Cinergy Health and primary care internist in New York.

"Having pets can be safe for you, your family and the pet if you do your homework carefully beforehand – learning about the specific types of pet, potential risks, how to prevent health problems," she says.

Read on to learn how to avoid getting 6 pet illnesses:

1.Toxoplasmosis

What it is: One of the most common parasitic diseases. It's caused by a microscopic critter called Toxoplasma gondii.

How you get it: Cats who eat infected birds, rodents and other small animals pass the parasites' eggs in their feces.

When you clean the litter box or do gardening where cats roam, you can accidently ingest infected feces, says veterinarian Eileen Ng, BVMS, of Western Veterinary Group in Lomita, Calif.

Kids face additional risk if they play in sandboxes that cats use as a bathroom.

You – and your cat – can also get toxoplasmosis by eating uncooked meats (such as lamb, pork or beef) from an infected animal, Ng says.

In pets: Cats usually don't show obvious symptoms, Ng says. It rarely causes significant medical problems in healthy animals.

But some may have fever, vomiting or diarrhea.

If so, ask your vet to do a blood test for toxoplasmosis. It's treated with antibiotics, such as clindamycin, and drugs that prevent the parasite from reproducing.

There's no vaccine.

In humans: Most healthy adults don't develop a serious illness from toxoplasmosis. They may not even know they have it, says Janet Horn, M.D., Lifescript women's health expert.

Symptoms, if noticed at all, are similar to the flu or mononucleosis: severe fatigue, muscle aches, swollen lymph nodes and blurred or reduced vision, eye pain and redness.

They can last a month or more but go away without treatment, she says.

For young children, the elderly or anyone with a weakened

immune system, toxoplasmosis is dangerous: When your body can't fight the parasite, it damages the brain, eyes and other organs.

Pregnant women may also pass the disease to babies. Even if the parasite is dormant in the mother, it continues to live in her tissue and can cross the placenta to infect the fetus.

"Most infants infected in the womb are born with no symptoms. But they can develop them later in childhood. A few can be born with brain or eye damage," Horn says.

Because of these risks, it's standard practice to test pregnant women for toxoplasmosis.

Doctors may treat the parasite with antibiotics pyramethamine and sulfadiazine.

Protect yourself:
- Clean the litter box daily.
- If you're pregnant or immune-suppressed, have someone else clean it.
- Wear gloves when cleaning the litter box or gardening. Wash hands thoroughly afterwards.
- Keep your cat indoors to reduce exposure risk.
- Don't feed cats raw meat.
- Keep kids' sandboxes covered.

2. Ringworm

What it is: Ringworm is a fungal infection, not an actual worm, Ng says.

How you get it: Petting an infected animal, most commonly a cat.

"It can go either way," Ng notes. "You can give an animal ringworm, or they can give it to you."

Pets typically get ringworms through contact with an infected animal. People pass it by touching an infected person's skin or contaminated items like unwashed clothing, shower surfaces and combs, according to the Centers for Disease Control and Prevention (CDC).

In pets: Fur loss is common, because the infection damages hair follicles. This is often the only sign of infection, Ng says.

Vets check for ringworm using a black light. If fur glows green, Fluffy has it. Even if the black-light test is negative, they'll do a fungal culture to double-check.

Topical shampoo can help, but oral antifungal medication is the best treatment, Ng says.

In humans: It causes a ring-like patch on your scalp or skin, says <u>Robin Miller</u>, M.D., Lifescript women's health expert.

Skin patches are itchy, raised and have sharply defined red edges. On the scalp, it shows up as bald spots. And it leaves nails discolored, thick and crumbly.

Skin ringworm shows up 4-10 days after contact and is treated with over-the-counter antifungal cream or pills containing clotrimazole.

Scalp ringworm usually takes 10-14 days and you'll need to see a doctor for treatment.

Protect yourself:
- See your doctor and vet immediately if you or your pet have symptoms.
- Bleach all bedding your cat has been on to kill fungus.
- Clean all surfaces Fluffy has touched with diluted bleach.

3. Roundworm

What it is: Unlike ringworm, roundworm actually is a worm - an intestinal parasite.

How you get it: Accidently ingesting cat or dog feces. How? By petting an infected animal that licks its backside and then its coat.

In pets: If stool contains what looks like spaghetti, ask the vet to test a fecal sample for eggs, Ng says.

If found, an oral dewormer medication can kill them. Go back for a retest to make sure worms are gone.

In humans: If you swallow worm eggs, they hatch in your intestine, Miller explains.

Hatched eggs can migrate to the throat and enter lungs, where they're coughed up and re-swallowed. Eggs then land back in the intestine, where they grow, reproduce and release more eggs.

In many people, this disease has few or no symptoms. But it can resemble pneumonia, particularly in the elderly or those with compromised immunity.

Within 2-3 months, roundworm can also cause severe abdominal pain, vomiting, fatigue, restlessness and disturbed sleep.

If you have it, you'll find eggs and/or worms in your stool, or, in severe cases, coming out of your nostrils, Miller says.

Fortunately, the infection can be cleared up with anthelmintics, medicine that kills the worms. In rare, severe cases, worms cause intestinal blockages requiring surgery to repair.

Protect yourself:
- Don't let infected pets lick you or your children.
- Wash hands after petting an animal.

- Deworm your pet regularly – the vet can prescribe a topical or oral dewormer.
- Keep your pet from eating other animals' feces.
- Test new puppies and kittens.

4. Giardia

What it is: A microscopic parasite that causes gastrointestinal problems.

How you get it: If you accidently swallow giardia (jee-AR-dee-uh) picked up from pet objects (like a toy or leash) contaminated with feces from an infected dog.

Dogs ingest eggs by eating another animal's feces or licking that dog's backside.

Once an animal or person has been infected, the parasite lives in the intestine and is passed through the feces. It can survive outside the body up to several months.

In pets: Giardia typically causes diarrhea in dogs, but they might not show symptoms, Ng says. Your vet will test a fecal sample for giardia eggs. If positive, it's treated with oral dewormer medication.

In humans: Although some people don't show any symptoms, most will have diarrhea, greasy stools, abdominal cramping, gas, nausea and a poor appetite.

Symptoms usually last up to six weeks, Horn says. If longer, they can lead to dehydration and weight loss.

Several prescription antibiotics, including metronidozole (Flagyl), are available to kill these parasites.

Protect yourself:

- Wash hands after handling animals and their toys, leashes or feces.

- Wear gloves when cleaning up after your pet.

- Dispose of feces right away so pets can't reinfect themselves.

5. Salmonella

What it is: A bacterial disease commonly associated with improperly cooked chicken, but you can get it from living reptiles too.

How you get it: By handling a turtle, tortoise, iguana, snake or lizard. It's transmitted though reptile feces, and the bacterium clings to clothing and skin.

In pets: Salmonella occurs naturally in many reptiles and doesn't usually make them sick. No salmonella treatment is typically needed, Ng says.

In humans: Symptoms last about a week and include diarrhea, fever and stomach pain.

"Salmonella [usually] resolves on its own and rarely requires antibiotic treatment," Miller says.

However, if it spreads from intestines to other organs, antibiotics *are* required or the disease can be deadly.

Protect yourself:
- Wash hands with soap and water immediately after handling a reptile.

- Wash clothing that has came into contact with them.

- Don't allow reptiles to roam the house freely.

- Keep reptiles out of the kitchen.
- Disinfect surfaces using diluted bleach or the disinfectant Roccal-D (available at vets' offices and online).

6. Rabies

What it is: A viral disease in mammals.

Thanks to widespread vaccination, it's extremely rare in house pets. Only 1% of cats and 0.3% of dogs tested positive for rabies in 2008, according to the CDC. Wild animals accounted for 93% of reported rabies cases.

How you get it: Through a bite from an infected animal, or less commonly, from a lick on an open cut.

In pets: Initial signs include excessive salivating and unusually aggressive behavior, says Ng.

When the rabies virus overtakes the animal's nervous system in 10-14 days, they can lose the ability to eat or drink. Death occurs soon after.

Animals suspected of having rabies may be quarantined for 10-14 days (to see if they survive).

Rabies isn't treatable in animals, so euthanasia is the only option after infection has occurred.

The only definitive diagnosis comes after death by testing a frozen section of the brain.

In humans: Rabies doesn't usually cause symptoms until late in the disease, by which time the prognosis is grim, Horn says.

When they do occur, symptoms include fever, headache, confusion, anxiety, difficulty swallowing and insomnia.

If you're bitten by a rabid animal, get medical attention right away. Starting a month-long series of shots immediately after exposure prevents the virus from taking hold in the body.

If infection sets in, there's no treatment. "Except in a small number of cases, the disease is fatal," Horn says.

Protect yourself:
- Vaccinate dogs, cats and ferrets.

- Get a pre-exposure shot if you work with animals or travel in undeveloped parts of the world where rabies is common.

Are You Pet Ready?

Undaunted by the above information? Is your family ready to bring home a new puppy, kitten or rescue animal? }

Patients do get labeled with a known diagnosis, why... because otherwise you don't get paid. Most of the patients have insurances, so you have to justify the lesions and something that is already known and something that is acceptable to the peers.

Reported by Elsevier & Elselvier;
- Pruritic response to infestation of human mite *Sarcoptes scabiei*. Severely itchy lesions typically present as small papules with noticeable curvy or straight burrows commonly located in skin folds, axillae, feet, thighs, elbows, genitalia, buttocks, breast areola and nipple, penis and scrotum, and interdigital web spaces

- Highly contagious in intimate or close personal contact; most commonly acquired by close contact with infected bedding, clothing, sexual relations, bedsharing, and handshaking

- Secondary signs may include general rash, urticaria, eczema, excoriation, and impetigo
- Patients may be asymptomatic for the first 2-4 weeks of infestation
- Permethrin is the treatment of choice for scabies

Synonyms
- Seven-year itch
- Sarcoptic itch
- Sarcoptes scabiei infection

Urgent action

Immunocompromised patients with Norwegian scabies may have exceedingly high numbers of parasites on the skin. These patients are highly infectious. Such patients should be placed in contact isolation and treated effectively to avoid widespread transmission to others.

Background

Cardinal features
- Primary lesions are extremely itchy, more severe at night, and present as small papules with noticeable curvy or straight burrows commonly located in skin folds, axillae, feet, thighs, elbows, genitalia, buttocks, breast areola and nipple, penis and scrotum, and interdigital web spaces
- Secondary lesions may also be present and result from scratching or infection
- Elderly, immunocompromised, and <u>Down syndrome</u> patients may present with severe

infestation of widespread and crusty lesions (Norwegian scabies)

- Alternatively, elderly patients may experience fewer lesions than younger adults, but with more itching

- Pediatric patients experience widespread bodily involvement more often than adults, including head, neck, and face involvement, which is unusual in adults

- <u>Permethrin 5% cream</u> is the preferred treatment for scabies, but <u>lindane 1% lotion</u> and <u>ivermectin</u> are alternative therapies

- Institutional scabies is common in nursing care facilities

Causes

Common causes

- Infestation with the human mite *Sarcoptes scabiei*

- Close or direct skin-to-skin contact, sharing unwashed garments, sexual relations, or bedsharing with an infected individual

- Poor (crowded, unsanitary) living conditions or institutional infection

Rare causes

Infestation from dog mite *S. scabiei* var. *canine*; however, burrows are not associated with this type of infestation as these mites cannot complete a life cycle in humans.

Serious causes

Norwegian, or crusted scabies, is caused by heavy infections of

S. scabiei in immunocompromised hosts, <u>AIDS</u>, elderly, and institutionalized patients.

Contributory or predisposing factors
Poverty, crowding, immunocompromised states, displaced populations, war refugees, closed institutions.

Epidemiology
Incidence and prevalence

Incidence
Precise statistics are unavailable; incidence may vary worldwide by 30-year cycles. Studies vary from 1-15 cases per 1000 people per year. Increased incidence during wars, famine, and social upheaval.

Prevalence
Variable, with greatest prevalence in institutionalized patients, conditions of poverty, displaced populations, refugees, migrant workers, and crowded conditions.

Frequency
Precise statistics unavailable. A worldwide ectoparasite. Some studies suggest 6-27% of general population has scabies, but other surveys find lower prevalence.

Demographics
Race
Occurs in all races, but may be seen less frequently in African-Americans (although some studies dispute this).

Socioeconomic status
Poor populations living in crowded conditions (e.g. refugees) have a higher frequency of scabies.

Codes
ICD-9 code
133.0 Scabies

Diagnosis
Clinical presentation
Symptoms
Intense nocturnal pruritus within 1-4 weeks after infestation.

Signs
- Inflamed, crusty lesions within 1-4 weeks after infestation in skin folds, axillae, feet, thighs, elbows, genitalia, buttocks, breast areola and nipple, penis and scrotum, and interdigital web spaces

- Linear or curvy burrows

- A 'wake sign' is the pattern of skin that may be seen on the palms of patients infected with scabies. It resembles the shape of a 'wake' left on the surface of water by a moving ship. It can be seen by the naked eye and is very specific for scabies

- Extensive involvement may be associated with secondary bacterial infection, scaling, and erythema

Associated disorders
AIDS, other immunocompromised states, Down syndrome, and institutionalized patients are more likely to acquire Norwegian scabies.

Differential diagnosis
Pediculosis

<u>Pediculosis</u> (head lice) is a common infestation among children. Lice are transmitted through contact (e.g. clothing, hairbrushes). They are usually confined to the scalp, but may be in the eyebrows and lashes.

Features
- Lice infestation
- Pruritic response
- Lymphadenopathy
- Itching

Atopic dermatitis

<u>Atopic dermatitis</u> (eczema) is an inflammation of the skin.

Features
- Eczematous response, particularly on the palms of hands and soles of feet
- Pruritic lesions or eruptions
- Itching

Seborrheic dermatitis

<u>Seborrheic dermatitis</u> is a skin disorder affecting the hairy areas of the body.

Features
- Scaling
- Erythema in hairy body regions

Dermatitis herpetiformis

Dermatitis herpetiformis is a rare skin rash that is caused

by an allergy to gluten and is often associated with celiac disease.

Features
- Intense pruritus in the extremities, often symmetrical and sometimes with a burning or stinging feeling
- Watery blisters that resemble pimples

Contact dermatitis

Contact dermatitis is a skin inflammation caused by an allergy or irritant (e.g. poison ivy, nickel compounds, cosmetics, drugs).

Features
- Eczematous response to environmental irritant
- Pruritic lesions or eruptions
- Itching

Nummular eczema

A coin-shaped skin rash that appears on the arms and legs. It usually clears up permanently on its own.

Features
- Itching
- Patchy erythematous plaques
- Distribution to sites of frequent itching; arms, pretibial area
- No burrows of scabies

Syphilis

Syphilis is a sexually transmitted disease.

Features
- Papulosquamous reaction on trunk, chest
- Fever, lymphadenitis
- Positive serologic test for syphilis
- No burrows of scabies

Other insect infestations

The bites of certain insects (e.g. chiggers, fleas, mosquitos, spiders) can produce red, itchy sores.

Features
- Papular urticaria at bite sites
- No burrows of scabies

Workup

Diagnostic decision
- Clinical presentation of scabies is characteristic but varies, depending on the duration and degree of infestation
- Clinical observation of the lesions and associated burrows in combination with microscopic determination of mites, eggs, and/ or feces is usually the only requirement for accurate diagnosis
- Entodermoscopy using a dermatoscope to render the skin surface translucent is a substitute for *ex vivo* microscopy. Dermoscopy allows identification of the scabies mite and its feces with equal sensitivity compared with *ex vivo* microscopy of burrow scrapings

- Consider other diagnostic possibilities if scabies is suspected but not confirmed by scraping

Guidelines
- Workowski KA, Berman SM; Centers for Disease Control and Prevention. <u>Sexually transmitted diseases treatment guidelines, 2006</u>. MMWR Recomm Rep 2006;55(RR-11):1-94. See section on <u>Scabies</u>

- Clinical Effectiveness Group, <u>British Association for Sexual Health and HIV (BASHH)</u>. <u>United Kingdom national guideline for the management of scabies infestation</u>. London (UK): British Association for Sexual Health and HIV (BASHH); 2008. Available at the <u>National Guideline Clearinghouse</u>

The <u>American Academy of Family Physicians</u> has produced the following document which discusses the diagnosis and management of scabies:
- Flinders DC, de Schweinitz P. <u>Pediculosis and scabies</u>. Am Fam Physician 2004;69:341-8

Don't miss!
- Pediatric patients may have vesicles on the palms and soles, eczema, impetigo, and nodular lesions

- Elderly patients may have fewer lesions than younger adults with more intense itching

- Norwegian scabies, a more severe infestation, is found in elderly, immunocompromised, or <u>Down syndrome</u> patients. It is associated with hand and/or feet involvement, crusty lesions rather than inflammatory papules or vesicles, excessive keratosis, nail dystrophy, wart-like formations on digits and trauma sites, gray or thick scales on the trunk of the body or the extremities, facial skin desquamation, hair shedding

Questions to ask

Presenting condition

- **Have you been in close contact with someone who has scabies?** Scabies is a highly contagious disease and can be transferred from one person to another very easily when in close contact

- **How long have you been experiencing the itching?** Incubation appears to be 1-4 weeks, and most patients are asymptomatic during that time

- **Does scratching the itch provide relief?** Destruction of the burrows by scratching can remove mites for a period of time, but not the eggs

- **Have you seen any linear or curved burrows anywhere on your body?** Burrows are indicative of mite infestation

- **Have you seen any vesicles with clear fluid?** Serous-filled vesicles are another classic characteristic of scabies

- **Where have you observed the lesions?** The lesions of scabies are commonly located in skin folds, axillae, feet, thighs, elbows, genitalia, buttocks, breast areola and nipple, penis and scrotum, and interdigital web spaces

- **Have you tried any medication for the lesions and, if so, what?** Topical steroids provide relief and suppress the inflammation; therefore, it is important to know if the patient has been treating the lesions for accurate diagnosis

Contributory or predisposing factors

Is there a history of predisposing factors? Close human contact, poor hygiene, animal contact (animal mites will attempt to feed on humans but will not survive; mite infestations are species specific).

Family history

Does anyone else in the family have these same symptoms or similar itching problems? This is a highly contagious disease and frequently involves family members.

Examination

- Check the skin folds and axillae, feet, thighs, elbows, genitalia, buttocks, breast areola and nipple, penis and scrotum, and interdigital web spaces for characteristic burrows

- Check the patient's skin for characteristic symptoms that are being attributed to an insect bite or dry, itchy skin

- Check the temporal pattern of itching; nocturnal pruritus is a general characteristic of scabies

- Check for serous-filled vesicles; scabies is associated with serous-filled vesicles rather than purulent-filled vesicles

- Check for secondary lesions (pinpoint erosions), pustules, scaling, erythema, and eczematous inflammation; these signs result from infection or excessive scratching

Summary of tests

- <u>Microscopic examination of skin scrapings</u> from the infected area for mites, feces, and/or eggs by mineral oil or potassium hydroxide preparation is the only diagnostic test required

- A skin biopsy will be diagnostic if the mite and/or its eggs are identified. The biopsy will show a type IV hypersensitivity reaction in the skin (inexpensive but may be time consuming). Finding the adult female mite is diagnostic, but it may not be readily apparent, especially with light infestations

- <u>Entodermoscopy</u> using a dermatoscope to render the skin surface translucent is a substitute for *ex vivo* microscopy. Dermoscopy allows identification of the scabies mite and its feces with equal sensitivity compared with *ex vivo* microscopy of burrow scrapings

Order of tests

- <u>Microscopic examination of skin scrapings</u>

- <u>Entodermoscopy of skin surface at the site of a burrow</u>

Tests

Other tests

<u>Microscopic examination of skin scrapings</u>

Description

Collect a skin sample from the infected area by scraping or shaving the area with a scalpel until pinpoint bleeding occurs.

Advantages/disadvantages
Advantage: microscopy is a simple and accurate method of analyzing the patient for mite infestation as determined by the presence of mites, eggs, egg casings, and/or fecal matter.

Normal
- No mites, eggs, egg casings, and/or fecal matter observed.

Abnormal
- Mites, eggs, egg casings, and/or fecal matter observed
- Keep in mind the possibility of false-positive results

Cause of abnormal result
Scabies infection.

<u>Entodermoscopy of skin surface at the site of a burrow</u>

Description
A hand-held epiluminescent stereomicroscope (dermatoscope) is used to view skin lesions. Dermoscopy renders the skin surface translucent and allows visualization of submacroscopic structures located in the epidermis and upper dermis.

Advantages/disadvantages
Advantage: dermoscopy is a simple, noninvasive method of analyzing the patient for mite infestation as determined by the presence of mites and/or fecal matter.

Normal

No mites or fecal matter observed.

Abnormal

- Mites or fecal matter observed
- Keep in mind the possibility of false-positive results

Cause of abnormal result

Scabies infection.

Clinical pearls

- A small drop of ink from a fountain pen dropped in the suspected burrow will be picked up by the burrow by capillary action. The ink will stop at the site of the female adult mite. This can be a useful guide to the optimal site for skin scraping

- Wear gloves during the examination of suspected skin lesions to avoid acquisition of scabies

- Scabies is often considered a sexually transmitted disease, but this may not be entirely accurate. It is the close contact, rather than the sexual act itself, that transmits scabies

- Scabies is not efficiently transmitted in school, offices, and other casual contact settings. Room-mates (particularly those who share bed linen and clothing), household contacts, and intimate partners efficiently spread scabies to each other

- Scabies mites can survive for 48-72h off the human body (in clothing, towels, other fomites). These items are potentially infectious to others if not properly cleaned. Wash all linen, clothing, and towels in the hot cycle of the clothes washer. Furniture (e.g. chairs, mattresses) should be cleaned, preferably with an antiseptic-scabicide solution

- It is often desirable to treat all family members simultaneously to avoid reinfection and intrafamily spread

Treatment

Goals
- Provide symptomatic relief
- Resolve mite infestation
- Prevent recurrence

Immediate action
Infection control is important to avoid spread to other susceptible individuals. This is particularly true in an institutional setting.

Therapeutic options

Summary of therapies
- First-choice treatment is <u>permethrin</u>.
  Permethrin is superior to topical lindane or oral ivermectin in reducing treatment failures and in decreasing itch. Permethrin may be used safely in pregnant women and pediatric patients

- The second-choice options include <u>ivermectin</u> or <u>lindane</u>. Ivermectin is the only oral scabicide, but it is expensive. Lindane is equally effective but is associated with neurotoxicity

- In patients with eczematous inflammation and pyoderma, signs of a secondary infection should be treated with appropriate antibiotics. A topical corticosteroid can be used to decrease inflammation before commencing scabicide treatment

- Persistent itching may be treated with oral antihistamines or topical antipruritic agents

- All patients should take appropriate <u>lifestyle</u> measures

- Norwegian scabies requires more aggressive treatment. It may be necessary to retreat these patients after 10-14 days to ensure eradication. In cases of hospitalized or institutionalized patients with Norwegian scabies, use contact isolation methods to prevent infection of other patients. This includes separate room, gloves, and gown during patient care activities; wash all linen in hot cycle of clothes washer, and treat bedding and pillows with scabicide before releasing the room to the next patient

Guidelines
- Workowski KA, Berman SM; Centers for Disease Control and Prevention. <u>Sexually transmitted diseases treatment guidelines, 2006</u>. MMWR Recomm Rep 2006;55(RR-11):1-94. See section on <u>Scabies</u>

- Strong M, Johnstone P. <u>Interventions for treating scabies (review)</u>. Cochrane Database Syst Rev. 2007, Issue 3: CD000320

- Clinical Effectiveness Group, <u>British Association for Sexual Health and HIV</u>

(BASHH). <u>United Kingdom national guideline for the management of scabies infestation</u>. London (UK): British Association for Sexual Health and HIV (BASHH); 2008. Available at the <u>National Guideline Clearinghouse</u>

The <u>American Academy of Family Physicians</u> has produced the following document which discusses the diagnosis and management of scabies:

- Flinders DC, de Schweinitz P. <u>Pediculosis and scabies</u>. Am Fam Physician 2004;69:341-8

- Fawcett R. <u>Ivermectin use in scabies</u>. Am Fam Physician 2003;68:1089-92

Order of therapies
- <u>Permethrin</u>
- <u>Ivermectin</u>
- <u>Lindane</u>
- <u>Lifestyle changes</u>

Efficacy of therapies
Scabies is generally eradicated successfully with one application of medication.

Medications and other therapies
Medications

<u>Permethrin [EBM]</u>
A scabicide used to eradicate mite infestations.

Dose
- Apply 5% cream from head to toe and leave on for 8-14h

- Wash off with water
- Repeat in one week, if necessary

Efficacy
Rates of 91% complete resolution have been reported.

Risks/benefits
Risk:
- Itching may increase temporarily after treatment

Benefits:
- Can be used in pregnant women and in infants older than 2 months
- Usually requires only one treatment

Side-effects and adverse effects
- Edema
- Numbness
- Pruritus
- Rash
- Tingling
- Transient burning
- Transient erythema

Contraindications
- No absolute contraindications reported
- Use with caution in children under 2 months

Evidence
- A Cochrane review compared various treatments for scabies and found that topical permethrin and benzyl benzoate was both

more effective than oral ivermectin, and oral ivermectin was more effective than lindane in curing scabies [1]*Level A*

[1]

Acceptability to patient
- This cream is more cosmetically acceptable than the other treatments
- Poorly absorbed; therefore, less likely to cause toxicity
- Usually effective with just one application

Follow-up plan
Repeat treatment in one week (no sooner), if necessary.

Patient and caregiver information
- All contacts must be treated
- Affected clothing and bedding must be washed in hot water immediately

Ivermectin [EBM]
This drug is an antihelminthic and is used to kill susceptible organisms. This is an off-label indication.

Dose
Oral:
- 200mcg/kg/dose as a single dose; may repeat dose in two weeks

Risks/benefits
Benefit: associated with rapid eradication of mites, which can induce systemic or ocular inflammation.

Side-effects and adverse effects
- Anorexia
- Constipation
- Diarrhea
- Dizziness
- Fatigue
- Fever
- Increased transaminase levels
- Leukopenia
- Nausea
- Pruritus
- Rash
- Somnolence
- Tremor
- Urticaria
- Vertigo

Contraindications
Pregnant women.

Evidence
- A Cochrane review compared various treatments for scabies and found that topical permethrin and benzyl benzoate was both more effective than oral ivermectin, and oral ivermectin was more effective than lindane in curing scabies [1]*Level A*
- Another small RCT in this review suggests there is no difference in clinical cure rates at 30 days between ivermectin and benzyl benzoate,

but the reviewers note that this trial is too small
to demonstrate an effect conclusively [[2]]*Level
B*

- A subsequent RCT, however, did find a
significantly greater cure rate at 30 days with
oral ivermectin compared with benzyl benzoate
[[3]]*Level A*

- An RCT comparing the use of lindane with oral
ivermectin found similar cure rates at 15 days
with both treatments [[4]]*Level A*

- However, a subsequent RCT found that
although the effects of topical lindane and oral
ivermectin were similar at 2 weeks, ivermectin
produced significantly greater cure rates at 4
weeks [[5]]*Level A*

[[2], [3], [4], [5]][1]
plan
Monitor patient for inflammatory responses.

Patient and caregiver information
- All contacts must be treated

- Affected clothing and bedding must be washed
in hot water immediately

Lindane [EBM]
This drug is a scabicide used to eradicate mite infestations.

Dose
- Apply 1% lotion from chin to toes and leave on
for 8-12h

- Wash off after 12h

- Repeat treatment in one week

- Apply lotion to head in children and leave on for 6-8h
- Trim fingernails

Efficacy
Highly effective.

Risks/benefits
Risks:
- Not recommended for use in pregnant women or young children
- Associated with neurotoxicity
- Excreted in breast milk
- Do not administer after bathing as this medication is readily absorbed and has an increased potential for toxicity

Side-effects and adverse effects
- Dizziness
- Eczematous eruptions
- Seizures
- Stimulation

Contraindications
- History of seizure disorders
- Pregnant women
- Premature infants
- Young children

Evidence

- A Cochrane review compared various treatments for scabies and found that topical permethrin and benzyl benzoate was both more effective than oral ivermectin, and oral ivermectin was more effective than lindane in curing scabies [1]*Level A*

- An RCT comparing the use of lindane with oral ivermectin found similar cure rates at 15 days with both treatments [[4]]*Level A*

- However, a subsequent RCT found that although the effects of topical lindane and oral ivermectin were similar at 14 days, the cure rates were significantly lower at 28 days with lindane compared with ivermectin [[5]]*Level A*

[[4], [5]][1]

Acceptability to patient
This medication may not relieve the itching and pruritus associated with scabies for up to 2 weeks after treatment.

Follow-up plan
Repeat treatment in one week.

Patient and caregiver information
- All contacts must be treated
- Affected clothing and bedding must be washed in hot water immediately

Lifestyle

Lifestyle changes
Avoid sharing linen, clothes, towels; choose bed mates carefully.

Summary of evidence

Evidence
- A Cochrane review compared various treatments for scabies and found that topical permethrin and benzyl benzoate was both more effective than oral ivermectin, and oral ivermectin was more effective than lindane in curing scabies [1]*Level A*

[1]

Clinical pearls
- If multiple members of family or communal living setting (e.g. apartments, dormitories) are infested, it is desirable to treat all members of the household simultaneously

- Single, sporadic cases may be treated individually

- Post-treatment itching is very common, secondary to delayed hypersensitivity to egg, mite antigens; this does not indicate treatment failure. Diffuse pruritus may also be psychogenic in origin; patients need advice, reassurance, and antipruritics as needed

- True treatment failures secondary to scabicide-resistant *S. scabiei* occur but are very uncommon. Treatment failures deserve referral to a dermatologist

Management in special circumstances
- For outbreaks in nursing homes or other communal living areas, a comprehensive approach becomes necessary. This includes mass screening of patients, staff, and support

personnel; information packet for staff, patients, and family; infection control measures (e.g. cleaning of linen, bed clothes, mattresses, pillows, chairs), and treatment for infected individuals

- In cases of hospitalized or institutionalized patients with Norwegian scabies, use contact isolation methods to prevent infection of other patients

Coexisting disease
- Patients who are immunocompromised (e.g. <u>HIV</u>-positive, elderly, and institutionalized patients) may require prolonged treatment to ensure nonrecurrence
- Treat patients who show signs of a secondary bacterial infection with an antistaphylococcal antibiotic

Special patient groups
Do not use lindane cream in pregnant women, young children, or premature infants due to the increased potential for neurotoxicity. Permethrin cream can be used in pregnant women and children who are at least 2 months old.

Patient satisfaction/lifestyle priorities
Good personal hygiene, and washing and maintaining separate clothing, towels, and beds are easy measures for most patients to take in addition to medication.

Patient and caregiver issues
Questions patients ask

- **Does a scabies infection mean I'm a 'dirty' person?** Educate the patient about the causes of scabies and assure them that poor hygiene is not the sole cause of infestation

- **How do I make sure this doesn't recur?** Educate the patient about the importance of treating all close contacts and cleaning all sources of mite habitation (e.g. bedding, clothes)

Health-seeking behavior

- **Has the patient waited too long before presenting?** Severe infestation can be the result of the patient waiting too long to seek proper medical treatment

- **Has the patient used any medication?** Use of topical or systemic corticosteroids can mask the characteristic symptoms of scabies, thereby making a quick, accurate diagnosis difficult

Follow-up

Plan for review
Monitor patients for eradication of mite infestation 7-14 days after treatment.

Information for patient or caregiver
- Educate patients that scabies is not a reflection of their personal hygiene

- Educate patients about the importance of treating all contacts and washing all bedding and clothing immediately

Ask for advice

Question 1
How contagious is scabies?

Answer 1
Scabies is transmitted by direct contact with skin or clothing of a person with an active infestation. It is not transmitted by casual contact, e.g. in an office setting.

Question 2
What is 'Norwegian' scabies?

Answer 2
A heavy infestation with scabies, often in immunocompromised or institutionalized patients. These patients may have thousands of mites on the skin and clothing. They often have thickened, lichenified skin folds from prolonged infection and itching. They are highly infectious to others, and they need to be isolated and vigorously treated.

Question 3
Can the mites from other animals cause scabies in humans?

Answer 3
No, but they can bite people and cause cutaneous reactions ('chiggers'). Only *Sarcoptes scabiei* are adapted to live for prolonged periods on human skin.

Question 4
Can the mite that causes human scabies survive in the environment unattached to humans?

Answer 4
Yes, but only for a short period of time (24-48h). They may survive in contaminated clothing, linen, or mattresses after

an infected person has been in contact with these materials. It is important to decontaminate the clothes, linen, and environment, as well as the patient with scabies, to prevent spread of infection to others.

Question 5
Can dogs be a source of symptoms of scabies in humans?

Answer 5
Occasionally; dog sarcoptic mange is due to *Sarcoptes scabiei* var. *canis*. Bites from dog scabies can cause symptoms of itching and papular urticaria in humans. Family outbreaks have occurred from dog mites. This form of scabies is not the same as human scabies due to a human-adapted form of mite known as *S. scabiei* var. *hominis*. Dog mites will not burrow in human skin and cannot complete their life cycle in humans. Eradication of dog mites will rapidly cure symptoms in families of dogs with mange.

Consider consult
Recalcitrant infestations, relapse.

Outcomes
Prognosis
Scabies is generally treated successfully with one application of medication.

Clinical pearls
- Persistent itch doesn't necessarily mean therapeutic failure. Transient worsening of itch may follow treatment as a hypersensitivity reaction to mite and egg fragments occurs
- Explain details of treatment carefully to avoid poor response

- Scaling or Norwegian scabies patients may benefit from a shower before treatment to improve permeability of skin to scabicide agent

Progression of disease

Therapeutic failure

In cases of incomplete resolution, treat patient again according to the manufacturer's recommendations.

Recurrence

- In case of recurrence, treat patient again according to the manufacturer's recommendations
- Recurrence is more common in cases of Norwegian scabies

Deterioration

Look for secondary bacterial infection, hypersensitivity reactions to the mite antigen, drug reactions, and drug resistance.

Clinical complications

- Some patients develop eczematous inflammation and pyoderma, which may become secondarily infected
- Persistent itching may be a problem in some patients
- Patients with persistent nodular lesions should be treated with intralesional steroids
- Referral to dermatologist advised

Consider consult

- Extensive secondary infection
- Outbreak settings

Prevention

Secondary prevention
- Treat all close contacts
- Wash clothing and bedding of infected people with hot water

Screening
Screening is not required, but all contacts of a patient should be treated.

Resources

References

Evidence references
[1] Strong M, Johnstone P. Interventions for treating scabies (review). Cochrane Database Syst Rev 2007, Issue 3: CD000320

[2] Glaizou P, Cartel JL, Alzieu P, et al. Comparison of ivermectin and benzyl benzoate for treatment of scabies. Trop Med Parasitol 1993;44:331-2 Abstract PubMed

[3] Nnoruka En, Agu CE. Successful treatment of scabies with oral ivermectin in Nigeria. Trop Doct 2001;31:15-8 Abstract PubMed

[4] Chouela EN, Abeldano AM, Pellerano O, et al. Equivalent therapeutic efficacy and safety of ivermectin and lindane in the treatment of human scabies. Arch Dermatol 1999;135:651-5 Abstract PubMed CrossRef

[5] Madan V, Jaskiran K, Gupta U, et al. Oral ivermectin in scabies patients: a comparison with 1% topical lindane lotion. J Dermatol 2001;28:481-4 Abstract PubMed

Guidelines

Workowski KA, Berman SM; Centers for Disease Control and Prevention. Sexually transmitted diseases treatment guidelines, 2006. MMWR Recomm Rep 2006;55(RR-11):1-94. See section on Scabies

Strong M, Johnstone P. Interventions for treating scabies (review). Cochrane Database Syst Rev. 2007, Issue 3: CD000320

Clinical Effectiveness Group, British Association for Sexual Health and HIV (BASHH). United Kingdom national guideline for the management of scabies infestation. London (UK): British Association for Sexual Health and HIV (BASHH); 2008. Available at the National Guideline Clearinghouse

The American Academy of Family Physicians has produced the following document which discusses the diagnosis and management of scabies:

Flinders DC, de Schweinitz P. Pediculosis and scabies. Am Fam Physician 2004;69:341-8

Fawcett R. Ivermectin use in scabies. Am Fam Physician 2003;68:1089-92

Further reading

Hicks MI, Elston DM. Scabies. Dermatol Ther 2009;22:279-92

Orion E, Marcos B, Davidovici B, Wolf R. Itch and scratch: scabies and pediculosis. Clin Dermatol 2006;24:168-75

Hengge UR, Currie BJ, Jager G, et al. Scabies: a ubiquitous neglected skin disease. Lancet Infect Dis 2006;6:769-79

Leone PA. Scabies and pediculosis pubis: an update of treatment regimens and general review. Clin Infect Dis 2007;44 Suppl 3:S153-9

Jacobson CC, Abel EA. Parasitic infestations. J Am Acad Dermatol 2007;56:1026-43

Dupuy A, Dehen L, Bourrat E, et al. Accuracy of standard dermoscopy for diagnosing scabies. J Am Acad Dermatol 2007;56:53-62

Usha V, Gopalakrishnan Nair TV. A comparative study of oral ivermectin and topical permethrin cream in the treatment of scabies. J Am Acad Dermatol 2000;42:236-40

Modamio P, Lastra CF, Sebarroja J, Marino EL. Stability of 5% permethrin cream used for scabies treatment. Ped Infect Dis J 2009;28(7):668

Zalaudek I, Giacomel J, Cabo H, et al. Entodermoscopy: a new tool for diagnosing skin infections and infestations. Dermatology 2008;216:14-23

Hu S, Bigby M. Treating scabies: results from an updated Cochrane Review. Arch Dermatol 2008;144(12):1638-41

Yoshizumi J, Harada T. "Wake sign": an important clue for the diagnosis of scabies. Clin Exp Dermatol 2008;34:711-4

Neynaber S, Wolff H. Diagnosis of scabies with dermoscopy. Can Med Assoc J 2008;178(12):1540-1

Associations
American Society of Microbiology
1752 N Street NW
Washington, DC 20036
Tel: (202) 737-3600
www.asm.org

Infectious Diseases Society of America
99 Canal Center Plaza, Suite 210
Alexandria, VA 22314
Tel: (703) 299-0200
Fax: (703) 299-0204
www.idsociety.org

Related topics

Contributors
Joseph Esherick, MD
Randolph L Pearson, MD
Steven M Opal, MD

[1] Strong M, Johnstone P. Interventions for treating scabies (review). Cochrane Database Syst Rev 2007, Issue 3: CD000320

[2] Glaizou P, Cartel JL, Alzieu P, et al. Comparison of ivermectin and benzyl benzoate for treatment of scabies. Trop Med Parasitol 1993;44:331-2 Abstract PubMed

[3] Nnoruka En, Agu CE. Successful treatment of scabies with oral ivermectin in Nigeria. Trop Doct 2001;31:15-8 Abstract PubMed

[4] Chouela EN, Abeldano AM, Pellerano O, et al. Equivalent therapeutic efficacy and safety of ivermectin and lindane in the treatment of human scabies. Arch Dermatol 1999;135:651-5 Abstract PubMed CrossRef

[5] Madan V, Jaskiran K, Gupta U, et al. Oral ivermectin in scabies patients: a comparison with 1% topical lindane lotion. J Dermatol 2001;28:481-4 Abstract PubMed

Associated disorders

- <u>Pediculosis</u>
- <u>Atopic dermatitis</u>
- <u>Seborrheic dermatitis</u>
- <u>Dermatitis herpetiformis</u>
- <u>Contact dermatitis</u>
- <u>Nummular eczema</u>
- <u>Syphilis</u>
- <u>Other insect infestations</u>

* Scabies - maybe resistant kind

** The patients get lesions with these classics entry and exit. But can parasites do that? Yes, you see a couple of pairs, hyper pigmentation. They get Koebner's phenomena.

Larva Migrans - most common diagnosis that I would use on a lot of Morgellon's patients because that's an acceptable diagnosis. A lot of symptoms are what the parasites do. It's a stage of parasites where the larva goes throughout the body and finds the destination or even come back to the bowel. Most of the worms will penetrate the bowels, into the bloodstream and some cases into the lungs.

I have a patient that had an x-ray and the result came out negative, however the patient is coughing and I can hear something from her lungs. I told my patients to bring me the x-ray film, and we could see small specks all over the x-ray. The patient is going through larva migrans with a pulmonary stage where it goes through the lungs.

These patients will sometimes tell me that they have chills in the night, sweats in the nights, fever it could be a night or a daytime, that's when they generate the larva. That is a pattern done by filaria, and is done in cycle. Other worms that can cause these symptoms are Tape Worm, Eccinococcus, Strongyloides, Schistosoma,

Roundworm, Ringworm, Hookworm, Pinworm, Toxocara

CHAPTER X
WHY DID I GET IT?

- Exposure - epidemiology, a lot of cases from Florida, Texas, California, states which are next to the water. These parasites act in a filaria form and one of the modes of transmissions is water. These larvae are migrating in the water, you go in the water, it penetrates and you get it. And also in places with warm or tropical climates.

** Why now it's happening not 10 years ago? More immigrants are coming from other parts of the world. Especially, third world countries brought parasites with them. Probably these parasites mutated to our environment and are now infecting places with tropical climate and also places that surrounded by water.

- Low Immunity - it could be any chronic illness or anybody in any medication

** I will check their immune system and I will find what is wrong with them by a series of test: immoglubin deficiency, B cell disorder, T cell disorder. Also, chronic disease likes diabetes, pulmonary diseases, HIV, Hepatitis. And autoimmune diseases

- Pets - whether it's being transmitted through mites, fleas.

** I have a patient who had a sick dog who was licking her, and now she had lesions all over her face. Another patient who used to sleep with her dog came back positive with dirofilaria, which is a dog hart worm. A lot of time people do not give anti-parasitic medicines to the dogs and in these warm climates the dogs and cats carry worms a lot and they have to be routinely treated.

- Travel - if you travel to a third world country where you were exposed. Example of the people was the militaries, missionaries. If you went to a place and eat something bad and got infected.

- Warm Climate

- Close Contacts - I have patient that I was treating that comes with her sister, now the sister got it, comes with her husband and now the husband got it. Close contacts were they're sharing foods, sleeping beds, using the same furniture's, and towels. The risk considering parasites are in different forms there's the egg, the larva and the adult. And, if it's a filariform there are two types, there is the larva form, which is actually infectious, it doesn't stay in the environment for long but on close contacts the larva form is still infectious you can get it. In the egg form it can stay in dirt, water.

- National Origin - if I see patients with different countries. I had a patient who came from Africa, South America and also one patient from Egypt. He apparently came in with a parasite, which is dormant, and these people have positive results. One of the patients from Africa actually has positive result for trichinella, but treating him for trichinella did not take the disease off, so he has this modified parasite that his harboring which is not being cured with any medication that is around.

CHAPTER XI
HOW DID I GET IT?

- Do you have a dog?
- Do you have a cat? - Who were sick and carrying worms
- Did you work in a pet store?
- Did you go out of the country?
- Did you eat something bad?
- Did you wash hand? - If your working in a high risk environment or if your cleaning your pet, and if the pet is infested with parasites there might be eggs in his body and your handling him, you put the eggs under your nails and you ingest them.
- Did you walk bare footed? - It could be in the beach, on the carpet where the dogs or cats has been there, the eggs or larva can penetrate your feet which can cause you the infection.

CHAPTER XII
WHAT CAN I DO ABOUT?

** It's a big blank. But, there's hope because patients do respond to certain regiments of treatments.

ANTI-PARASITICS
- Mebendazole
- Albendazole
- Ivermectin
- Kwell Lotion
- Permethrin
- Malathion
- Mebendazole Ointment

ANTIBIOTICS
- BACTRIM
- CIPRO
- DOXYCYLIN

- ZYVOX
- IV ANTIBIOTICS

** Also some for anti-fungal…aspergillus's, candida,

CHAPTER XIII
WHY NOW?

** Research that I started doing, which was accepted by American College Physicians for Presentation
DI-ETHYLCARBAMAZINE IN THE TREATMENT OF MORGELLON'S DISEASE

WHAT DO WE NEED?

- More research

- More money to do the research

- I need you help, to help you - any letters of support, or research grants would me appreciated

In United states this Medication is given only by CDC. And is not available for use by a regular doctor from a regular pharmacy. In other countries it is over the counter medication. So the disease is spreading for the failure of the access to treatment in this land of abundance.

CHAPTER XIV
QUESTIONS & ANSWERS

1) Is there a proven treatment that works for everyone?

No, every time I think that may have figured it out, the next patient will be entirely different. I get a treatment that some people respond beautifully to it, and then the next people wouldn't respond at all. That's makes it so hard, each individual case is a brand new thing. So far there's hasn't been anything that works for everyone. But we have some patients that are totally cured by certain treatments, but not everyone responds to these treatments.

2) If any placebo controlled studies done with any patients with Morgellon's, if any following classes of medicines: anti-bacterial, anti-fungal, anti-parasitic, anti-depressions and if not, are any such studies plan?

I think we were alluding to because each situation

maybe somewhat unique in terms of exposures to illnesses involved, genetically dispositions. Often treatments were individualized.

CHAPTER XV
DILEMMAS OF DIAGNOSIS OF
MORGELLON'S DISEASE

Strongyloides – cross reaction to strongylitis some patients have low positive reaction to Schistosoma.

echinococcus, is another test that comes out as low positive

- MRSA – (Methicillin-resistant staphylococcus aureus) detailed about the bacteriology that was presented, a lot of the times the lesion would be positive with MRSA and have not responded with any other antibiotic

Bacterial

- MRSA
- E- coli
- Pseudomonas
- Proteus

These Were seen these lesions, in my first opinion it was

a super infection because of the skin, and the second opinion that I have that a lot of these people will have a grand negative which is a bowel flora that is in the lesions.

** These bacteria were coming into the lesions because of the larva migrans from the bowel to the bloodstreams and into the lesions.

• Stool O & P – I sent out samples and when the results comes in its

Negative. So is the Urine,ANA, SED rate, ANCA. There may be low positive or borderline negative titers seen for Ankylostoma, Filaria, Dirofilaria.

DILEMMA OF THE LABORATORY DIAGNOSIS

The laboratories in America do not have technician well-trained in parasitology detection, especially in the commercial laboratories. The fresh stool needs to be examined in 48 hours, but you don't get the results until after a week. Hence, you get a test result that is negative. But the patient has the symptoms and the parasite; thus, the doctor calls the patient 'delusional', as there is no evidence to the patients' symptoms. And the patient does not get treated and one does not know what to treat the patient with. In a society of 'Evidence based Medicine' the doctor is trained to treat the evidence and not the patient. If the test is negative the Insurance company will not pay the doctor for treating the patient or pay for the medicines

CHAPTER XVI
PERSISTENCE OF INFECTION

Some patients will keep coming back with new lesions. The question then arises that is it a new lesion due to relapse, resistence or re-infection. It could be either one but a lot of times I believe it is re-infection. As the pet may be still infected or carrying the infection . or the pet may be re- infecting the household, the beds the couch, sofa etc. and the patient keeps getting re-infected. Or the pet is just continuing to shed egss. And the eggs can stay potent for a long time. Even on surfaces and beds and chairs leading to re-infections.

Concomitant bacterial Infections:

On several occasions there is concomitant bacterial Infections on th skin lesions,

These could be the skin flora of Staphylococcus epidermidis or aureus or MRSA. Or it could be an enteric pathogen that migrated with the larva of the parasite during the Larva Migrans phase. These are very commonly proteus sp.. They can also be enterococcus, pseudomonas, E.coli etc.

CHAPTER XVII
THE FIBERS

SITES OF SKIN LESIONS: The lesions very commonly occur initially at the site of the infection. Then the reside in the flexural areas of the body and keep recurring either as the residual infection or re- infection.

THE FIBER COLORS:
Patients see blue fibres which is known to be the shaft of the parasite in the venous phase. The look red in the arterial phase. The white fuzz that comes out is the excreta of the filamentous worms. The sand that comes out is the eggs of the worms. The patients feel it as nodules. Once they itch on it or expel the egg, it becomes an open micro sore evidencing the fact that it is a solid granule that comes out and not the pus as in acne.

The patients very commonly have a concomitant infection with disseminated Herpes Simplex, which is then superinfected with very commonly, MRSA or Proteus.

Most of these patients may also have immune – dysfunction or some other immune compromising disease states.

SOLUTIONS

Pet hygiene should be taken seriously. Consider home hygiene. Do special laundry care. Ther should be regular vaccuming and cleaning. Use Hot dryer. People should set limits with their pets. No sleeping until sure of the pet. Careful cuddling. Young children would be more vulnerable. So the parents need to keep an eye on their playing.Indoor litter bed should be avoided. De-worming of the pets should be done routinely with constant monitoring of your pets stools and regular vet checks. Any infested ares should be cleaned . Clothes and linen could be bleached. Carpets, if infested should be replaced.

RESOURCES

References
Evidence references

[1] Strong M, Johnstone P. Interventions for treating scabies (review). Cochrane Database Syst Rev 2007, Issue 3: CD000320

[2] Glaizou P, Cartel JL, Alzieu P, et al. Comparison of ivermectin and benzyl benzoate for treatment of scabies. Trop Med Parasitol 1993;44:331-2 Abstract PubMed

[3] Nnoruka En, Agu CE. Successful treatment of scabies with oral ivermectin in Nigeria. Trop Doct 2001;31:15-8 Abstract PubMed

[4] Chouela EN, Abeldano AM, Pellerano O, et al. Equivalent therapeutic efficacy and safety of ivermectin and lindane in the treatment of human scabies. Arch Dermatol 1999;135:651-5 Abstract PubMed CrossRef

[5] Madan V, Jaskiran K, Gupta U, et al. Oral ivermectin in scabies patients: a comparison with 1% topical lindane lotion. J Dermatol 2001;28:481-4 Abstract PubMed

Guidelines
Workowski KA, Berman SM; Centers for Disease Control

and Prevention. Sexually transmitted diseases treatment guidelines, 2006. MMWR Recomm Rep 2006;55(RR-11):1-94. See section on Scabies

Strong M, Johnstone P. Interventions for treating scabies (review). Cochrane Database Syst Rev. 2007, Issue 3: CD000320

Clinical Effectiveness Group, British Association for Sexual Health and HIV (BASHH). United Kingdom national guideline for the management of scabies infestation. London (UK): British Association for Sexual Health and HIV (BASHH); 2008. Available at the National Guideline Clearinghouse

The American Academy of Family Physicians has produced the following document which discusses the diagnosis and management of scabies:

Flinders DC, de Schweinitz P. Pediculosis and scabies. Am Fam Physician 2004;69:341-8

Fawcett R. Ivermectin use in scabies. Am Fam Physician 2003;68:1089-92

Further reading

Hicks MI, Elston DM. Scabies. Dermatol Ther 2009;22:279-92

Orion E, Marcos B, Davidovici B, Wolf R. Itch and scratch: scabies and pediculosis. Clin Dermatol 2006;24:168-75

Hengge UR, Currie BJ, Jager G, et al. Scabies: a ubiquitous neglected skin disease. Lancet Infect Dis 2006;6:769-79

Leone PA. Scabies and pediculosis pubis: an update of treatment regimens and general review. Clin Infect Dis 2007;44 Suppl 3:S153-9

Jacobson CC, Abel EA. Parasitic infestations. J Am Acad Dermatol 2007;56:1026-43

Dupuy A, Dehen L, Bourrat E, et al. Accuracy of standard dermoscopy for diagnosing scabies. J Am Acad Dermatol 2007;56:53-62

Usha V, Gopalakrishnan Nair TV. A comparative study of oral ivermectin and topical permethrin cream in the treatment of scabies. J Am Acad Dermatol 2000;42:236-40

Modamio P, Lastra CF, Sebarroja J, Marino EL. Stability of 5% permethrin cream used for scabies treatment. Ped Infect Dis J 2009;28(7):668

Zalaudek I, Giacomel J, Cabo H, et al. Entodermoscopy: a new tool for diagnosing skin infections and infestations. Dermatology 2008;216:14-23

Hu S, Bigby M. Treating scabies: results from an updated Cochrane Review. Arch Dermatol 2008;144(12):1638-41

Yoshizumi J, Harada T. "Wake sign": an important clue for the diagnosis of scabies. Clin Exp Dermatol 2008;34:711-4

Neynaber S, Wolff H. Diagnosis of scabies with dermoscopy. Can Med Assoc J 2008;178(12):1540-1

Associations

American Society of Microbiology
1752 N Street NW
Washington, DC 20036
Tel: (202) 737-3600
www.asm.org
Infectious Diseases Society of America
99 Canal Center Plaza, Suite 210
Alexandria, VA 22314
Tel: (703) 299-0200
Fax: (703) 299-0204

www.idsociety.org

Related topics

Contributors

Joseph Esherick, MD
Randolph L Pearson, MD
Steven M Opal, MD

[1] Strong M, Johnstone P. Interventions for treating scabies (review). Cochrane Database Syst Rev 2007, Issue 3: CD000320

[2] Glaizou P, Cartel JL, Alzieu P, et al. Comparison of ivermectin and benzyl benzoate for treatment of scabies. Trop Med Parasitol 1993;44:331-2
Abstract PubMed

[3] Nnoruka En, Agu CE. Successful treatment of scabies with oral ivermectin in Nigeria. Trop Doct 2001;31:15-8
Abstract PubMed

[4] Chouela EN, Abeldano AM, Pellerano O, et al. Equivalent therapeutic efficacy and safety of ivermectin and lindane in the treatment of human scabies. Arch Dermatol 1999;135:651-5
Abstract PubMed CrossRef

[5] Madan V, Jaskiran K, Gupta U, et al. Oral ivermectin in scabies patients: a comparison with 1% topical lindane lotion. J Dermatol 2001;28:481-4
Abstract PubMed

Last updated: 31 Dec 2009
Close

- Summary

- Description

- Synonyms

- Urgent action

- <u>Background</u>
- <u>Cardinal features</u>
- <u>Causes</u>
- <u>Common causes</u>
- <u>Rare causes</u>
- <u>Serious causes</u>
- <u>Contributory or predisposing factors</u>
- <u>Epidemiology</u>

PH.-(727)-547-5232
FAX-(727)-547-5233

1990 – Present: PRIVATE PRACTICE

TRAINING HISTORY:

- **1988-1990: PGY4&5:FELLOWSHIP:**
  INFECTIOUS DISEASE
  New York Hospital of Queens, Main street,
  Flushing, New York

- **1985-1987: PGY2&3:RESIDENCY:**
  INTERNAL MEDICINE
  Jersey city Medical Center, 50 Baldwin Ave.,
  Jersey City, NJ

- **1984-1985: PGY1: INTERNSHIP:**
  INTERNAL MEDICINE
  Methodist Hospital, 601, 5th Ave Brooklyn, NY

- **1978-1984: MEDICAL SCHOOL:** Bachelor
  of Medicine & Bachelor of Surgery
  Christian Medical College, India

QUALIFICATIONS:

- **ABIM : BOARD CERTIFICATION**
  -2: Infectious Disease: 1996-2006
- **ABIM: BOARD CERTIFICATION-1 :**
  Internal medicine: 1990-2000
- **ECFMG :1984**
- **M.B.B.S. :1984**

AWARDS AND HONORS:

- PHYSICIAN OF THE YEAR –2006 BY NRCC
- MADISON'S WHO'WHO
- STANFORD WHO'S WHO
- AMERICAN COLLEGE OF PHYSICIANS RESEARCH AWARD- FIRST PLACE-1990

MEMEBERSHIPS:

- AMERICAN COLLEGE OF PHYSICIANS
- INFECTIOUS DISEASE SOCEITY OF AMERICA
- FLORIDA INFECTIOUS DISEASE SOCEITY OF AMERICA
- AMERICAN MEDICAL ASSOCIATION
- FLORIDA MEDICAL ASSOCIATION
- PINELLAS COUNTY MEDICAL SOCEITY
- FLORIDA ASSOCIATION OF PHYSICIANS FROM INDIA

- AMERICAN ASSOCIATION OF PHYSICIANS FROM INDIA
- PINNELLAS PARK CHAMBER OF COMMERCE